I0759849

SØREN ULRIK THOMSEN

STORE KONGENSGADE 23

SØREN ULRIK THOMSEN

STORE KONGENSGADE 23

Translated by Hunter Simpson

ERIS

To Jane

ERIS

265 Riverside Drive
New York 10025

ISBN 978-1-967751-10-5

CONTENTS

Suddenly, in my helpless rage, I felt an urge to write something about my mother.

Peter Handke, ***A Sorrow Beyond Dreams***

1

On 14 March, shortly after midnight, my mother died. The time has come to revisit Store Kongensgade 23.

2

Is there a single year or place in a person's life that, as time passes, will reveal itself to have been the most important? The point at which the compass needle should be placed, because everything before was oriented, dreamlike, toward it, and everything after reflects back at this center, the meaning of which, of course, one cannot perceive until much later?

Yes, there is, and you don't have to speak with a person for very long before you can home in on the time and place of this strange nucleus in their life. For as we grow older, we tell the same stories again and again, and here I too will tell a story that I've told (some of) before. But as the author I am also the text's first reader, so I do this in the hope that, as I tell the story, I may come to write something surprising even to myself, and therefore, perhaps, also worth reading for others.

And that's not the only reason, for why do we write at all? To ward off death, to win back a lover, to capture and immortalize moments that would otherwise be lost forever? Or perhaps, conversely, it's to unburden ourselves of other moments, in the hope that they won't haunt us for all eternity. To jettison our experiences, so that, with renewed ignorance, we may then tell the same story again.

In my case, the place is the fourth floor of Store Kongensgade 23, where my family moved from Stevns when my father, a banker, was hired at the head office of the Bikuben Savings Bank on Silkegade, and the time period begins on 12 August 1972 and stretches onward for a year. It was here, during my seventeenth and eighteenth years, that I experienced things so weighty that

I somehow can't remember them at all, and other things so wonderful that I can recall them in the sharpest detail. And though it's hardly unique to me that this magical unit of time and space, which ceaselessly draws my thoughts back to it, should have occurred during puberty (the time of change par excellence), it still astounds me that this single, distant year of my life has not been long overshadowed by any of the events of the fifty intense years that followed.

Yes, it astounds me, when I think back on the half-century when I met most of the people who've been truly significant to me, when my professional endeavors unfolded, when art and literature and music flowed through me, when thoughts arose and were pursued and guided to their conclusions, when I got married and divorced and the love of my youth died after many years of dreadful illness, when sudden inspirations razed my mind and swept my table clear (even as abiding insights were arriving as discreetly and distinctly as the sound of a drop hitting the kitchen sink), when romances and regrets, sex and friendships and dramatic feuds and travels around the world filled my days and dreams, when conversations braided themselves in and out of one another and continued and were interrupted and then resumed when we met again on a random Tuesday at Café Blå Time.

3

But before I tell my story from the beginning, I must give an account of an invitation I received from the Museum of Copenhagen, which in 2010 put on an exhibition about "new Copenhageners", a term that they used to encompass both immigrants from other countries and those who had moved to the city from Denmark's provinces, all of whom were asked to contribute the single object that defined for them the moment when they became a Copenhagener. I knew right away that my contribution would be the class photo of the tenth-grade students at Sølvgade School (1972–3), for here my face appears among those of the thirteen Copenhageners with whom I went to school, and of whom, as a newly established resident of Store Kongensgade 23, I was now one, a fact of which I, a child of the provinces, have always been excessively proud, joyful as I was and still am to this day to have been granted clemency and released from provincial life. But my copy of the photo taken by Danish School Photography was in awful condition, and it occurred to me to ask our old homeroom teacher, Bodil Ulrich, whether she still had her copy on hand.

Bodil must've been in her mid-thirties, which would make her around twenty years older than we students in the school's oldest class. Pretty, and with a faint, charming Norwegian accent, she was full of unprejudiced, youthful energy. While the heavy costumes of '70s youth comprised sheepskin coats, workman's shirts, and clunky leather boots, Bodil, with her slightly angled cat-eye glasses and her hair done up high, retained the far lighter and more elegant style of the '60s, and generation-wise she resided somewhere between us and our parents—younger and smarter than they were, yet still an adult, unlike us students, ravaged as we were by puberty and exhausted by schooling, with our insolent attitude deriving its legitimacy from the youth movement of the previous decade, even as we also (knowing full well that the welfare state would likely catch us) permitted ourselves an unheard-of and ostentatious idleness. True to their upbringing, the girls were dutiful and sweet, but the boys were heedlessly harsh and sarcastic toward one another. In that thoroughly politicized period of cultural upheaval, the tenth grade of Sølvgade School had its share of bohemians as well as aspiring bankers, and neither side spared the other from ridicule.

Though I clearly remember her sighing at our childishness, Bodil never took sides, but spoke to every single student with the same understanding and respect. When, fifteen years after our last day of school, she invited us to a reunion at her house in Gentofte, which was imbued with the same '60s stylishness as Bodil herself, it was obvious that every one of her former students, regardless of their behavior, had respected her and perhaps also, in all discretion, practically loved her, and it was touching to watch how we all sought her gracious and encouraging gaze, appealing to her compassion for our problems and her admiration for our achievements as, with blushing cheeks, we took turns telling her about the years that had passed and our dreams for the future.

The telephone book informed me that she now lived on Esthersvej in Hellerup, and my call was quickly answered by her husband, Jørgen. In his younger days, Jørgen Ulrich was a famous tennis player with many Danish championship titles to his name, and he once made it all the way to the quarterfinals at Wimbledon. In contrast to his avant-garde brother Torben, also a professional tennis player, Jørgen was decidedly bourgeois, a legal advisor and the director of an insurance company. Still, he too was wrapped in the aura of the enchanted '60s, and though I don't know how he and Bodil met, I like to imagine that it was out on the tennis courts, and that after the match, slim and beautiful and dressed all in white, rackets slung over their shoulders, they strolled through the summer evening to a place where, befitting of that stylish modernity, they could enjoy drinks and cigarettes ("to the sound of cool jazz" I almost wrote before thinking better of it, wanting to avoid the sort of excessively coherent historical set design at which film people so excel but which is rarely found in reality, filled as it always is with the wreckage of previous decades, and bearing only a few state-of-the-art elements: behind the low, minimalist, white leather sofa there will invariably rise an inherited grandfather clock).

I told him about the invitation from the Museum of Copenhagen and my hunt for the old class photo. "Unfortunately it won't be possible for you to speak with Bodil". Jørgen said; "she's had a stroke and she can't speak or move anymore, even though she's fully conscious somewhere in there". Petrified and wide awake, what a frightful thought. I sat down and composed a letter in which I explained to her how much she still meant to me, long after our one year at Sølvgade School. I sent the letter to Esthersvej along with my poetry collection *Hjemfalden* and asked Jørgen to take it to her in the hospital. Shortly after that came my fifty-fourth birthday, which Jørgen, who really didn't know me at all, must have seen in the newspaper's long list of people born on 8 May, because on my answering machine he left a touching and sincere message wishing me a happy birthday and warmly thanking me for the letter and the beautiful poems, which Bodil was very pleased to receive.

Two months later, the newspaper reported that Jørgen Ulrich had died while traveling in Greece, age seventy-four. The past was beginning to fall away. Right in front of me.

4

What I remember first and foremost about Store Kongensgade 23 is the whirring feeling that *now* the future could begin, and every time I revisit the address the sight of it fills me with an intense, intoxicating expectation of a time yet to come, as if this house where I lived, now almost fifty years ago, were a mysterious incarnation of the place from which all future will forever radiate, though the house itself belongs to the past.

Life without expectations must be impossible, and in recent years I've come to understand how every one of our deeds, thoughts, and feelings, though they unquestionably transpire in a shimmering present and are unthinkable without the preconditions of the past, are oriented, dreamlike, toward the future, like leaves toward the sun. When, at the age of sixty, I was divorced from my wife, one of my greatest sorrows was that our shared future now belonged to the past, because the pleasure of walking hand in hand down Willemoesgade on a drizzly Tuesday afternoon in October was also the pleasure of knowing that we would do so again, and the enjoyment of mussels in saffron sauce and steak served with lemon slices at the tiny restaurant in the gray courtyard that cuts an odd L-shape into a neighborhood behind an Odeon cinema somewhere in Europe was intensified by the awareness that we would one day return to the same address, which in the meantime we would keep to ourselves, so that, like love, it would always be ready to resurrect itself for us alone.

Every book I read inspires me to read another, and every one of the words I'm writing now is written with a yearning for the next, the unwritten, which can only emerge through the act of writing. I found out what happens when this sense of expectancy cannot be mobilized one year ago when, following an orgasm, I saw bloody semen on the white sheet. Terrified, I called in the next morning and got an emergency appointment with a doctor who, though my urine and blood tests showed nothing concerning, recommended further urological examinations, which, owing to Christmas and a long waiting list, had to wait a whole month, during which time I undertook absolutely nothing apart from lying in my bed and staring at the wall, for though I no longer had any symptoms, it made no sense to lose myself in a piece of music, to eat dinner with a good friend, to read or write so much as a line, because, if I didn't know whether or not I'd soon be dead, then I couldn't meet my friend with the pleasure of knowing that we would meet again, and I could no longer read or write with the expectation that each line would be followed by another. However, as soon as I was able—thanks to a humiliating prostate examination and a painful cystoscopy—to abandon the idea that the bloody semen was caused by anything dangerous (it was instead likely the result of a burst blood vessel), the paused film jolted back into motion.

It's not only the knowledge that today will be followed by a new day, but also the expectation that the next day will be new in the sense of being better than the previous one, and perhaps even wonderful. This, I truly believe, is what keeps us alive. "Behold, I make all things new", said Christ (according to the Book of Revelation), and when I lose heart, I think of the wedding at Cana, where Christ saved the good wine for last. So perhaps even on my dying day I'll be able to look forward to the best of life, just as, on an August day in 1972 after a childhood in Stevns, I could lean out of the window on the fourth floor of Store Kongensgade 23 and, with a rejoicing heart, watch the sun reflecting off the chrome of the cars as traffic streamed endlessly down the street where my new life was to begin.

5

I never got to meet Ole Sarvig, whose poetry has been immeasurably important to me, because one week after his sixtieth birthday in November 1981 he killed himself by jumping out of a window. This has always seemed inexplicable to me, and when I've asked people who knew Sarvig, they have all had different accounts of his final, unhappy years, of which you can get a strong impression from his (in more ways than one) despairing psalms. They were all credible, and yet no one could really give me an answer, so when I met his longtime editor, the inimitably stylish Erik C. Lindgren, at a party recently, I asked him, too, if he knew why Sarvig did it. "I think", he said, "Sarvig felt that time had passed him by". And although time in 1981 was in a certain sense more attuned with Ole Sarvig than it had been for many years (because my generation revered his poetry, which suddenly seemed to speak to the atmosphere and aesthetics of the new decade, though unfortunately he probably never knew it), he himself was no longer attuned with this strange phenomenon, Time, which he had so masterfully captured almost forty years earlier when he stood upon "the bridge of the hours".

Lindgren's diagnosis seemed all the more convincing because it left me feeling uncomfortably exposed. For I, too, can feel time passing me by. When in the morning I lie swaying somewhere between wakefulness and sleep, I sense myself vacating the familiar—though not, for that reason, unproblematic—past that just enfolded me in dreams, as a barrage of cold little waves thrusts me into an alien present with which I am now so out of sync that I feel like an object of curiosity. On the whole, I understand the newspapers' write-ups and reviews of new books, exhibitions, and concerts just fine, but more and more references are unknown to me, and, conversely, it always comes as a shock when intelligent and well-informed people perhaps just fifteen years younger than I are bored to tears by Hitchcock's *Vertigo*, because, masterwork or not, it's simply too slow, or when they haven't heard of Lyndon B. Johnson, commissaire Maigret, or Dusty Springfield, all of whom are inextinguishable stars in my solar system.

Ole Sarvig had just turned sixty when he jumped out of a window, Tove Ditlevsen took her life at fifty-seven, while Frank Jæger was only fifty-one when he died of alcoholism. Time had passed them by, and as a sixty-five-year-old I've now lived longer than any of them, and every morning when I look in the mirror it's as if I'm seeing a phantom. Yes, I know, a bit rich coming from me, as I have always refused to countenance the grousing of grown men about turning fifty and losing their youth, telling them that I can't accept complaints about being granted a long life, because when I look back I see far too many people who died far too young: the love of my youth, Annemette, so brilliantly beautiful, bent over her restlessly ornamented pencil drawings, which she gradually lost sight of as she grew petrified with fear about her protracted illness; Michael, whom I ran into on Classensgade and spoke with superficially about everything but the chemotherapy that, I could plainly see, had left only a few hairs on his head; Majken, who called from Aarhus and told me that her whole body had suddenly turned yellow, and asked me to read some poems at her wedding, which she barely survived to see. And good-natured Svend from my village school with his chalk-white hair, who worked as a waiter alongside his mother and couldn't live out his homosexuality in their little rural world, but brought a certain virus home with him from a charter trip.

And when I look ahead, I see how plagued by acute as well as temporarily overcome illnesses those brave souls are, most of them, who are just ten years older than I, and as it isn't likely that things will progress any differently in my case, I live in this limbo like one whose sentencing has been postponed: grateful, but fearful of all the sour wine that must be consumed before the good wine is served.

6

I fear suddenly slumping down in a train seat on a Friday afternoon at one of the overground stations south of Copenhagen as the light from a nearby industrial kitchen burns through the November darkness.

But I also fear old age.

I fear the illnesses, the absurdities, and the overhead lighting on the linoleum hallways of the institutions that get a new name every ten years out of shame over the smell of excrement and chemicals that clings to the previous one: elderly home, nursing home, assisted living facility, senior housing.

I fear the little symptoms that, in their ambiguity, could be either harmless or fatal: the slight shortness of breath that can probably be blamed on the fact that you aren't what one would call an athlete, and isn't necessarily an early sign of emphysema; the stabbing pain that might be emanating from something lurking in your bones or festering in your stomach, but could also be caused by a cramped muscle or a pinched nerve (is that a thing?); the keys on the keyboard that you miss just a little too often; the kitchen utensils that slip out of your hands every now and then, which shouldn't immediately lead your thoughts straight to Parkinson's (runs in the family) but does all the same.

I fear the relatively mild condition in which you can manage to get by on your own—go shopping, pay the rent, and poke at your cell phone—even though a certain quantity of the thousands of threads that were painstakingly spun throughout your life between the aquarium of your inner world and the harsh reality beyond have now snapped, so that alongside your rational behaviors you emit a vague aura of oddness that causes others to take another look at you before quickly averting their eyes.

Just as I do myself when I suddenly spot him on the street after forty-five years—it is, without a doubt, the selfsame man from whom I sought help when I was young and baffled by the violent anxiety attacks that were making it impossible for me to live even a somewhat orderly life, because these attacks were visited upon me with total unpredictability and could only be pacified by my taking my clothes off and lying face down on a cold floor, where the disparity between the warmth of my skin and the cold of the floor would detach my body from everything else and momentarily establish me as an autonomous planet in the universe. But the constant expectation that my anxiety would soon strike again, combined with the uncertainty about when this would happen, completely robbed me of control over my life, whether in the present moment or in a week's time. What was the cause of this mysterious, paralyzing, ineffable anxiety? I must have thought that this man could tell me, though how I found him I can't recall—likely through an advertisement in which he called himself a psychoanalyst, which unfortunately remains a title without any official credentials, meaning that anyone who thinks they might like to be a psychoanalyst can simply call themself one. And that's exactly how I remember him, as "someone who would like to be a psychoanalyst", as he sat in his chair by the couch, in front of a bookshelf bearing the blue *Standard Edition* of Freud's *Complete Works*, with a strange, all-knowing, imperturbable, Buddhistic smile which imparted to me neither wisdom nor aid. And it is by this smile that I immediately recognize him, though he has since become an old man, curiously dressed in baggy second-hand clothes and a knitted hat slipping smurf-like over his left ear, while that eternal, unprompted smile hangs in front of his face, announcing the presence of a man who, in his later years, is not exactly crazy but is not all there either, and who, now far beyond the point at which he might have been reconciled with reality, seems to have wholly abandoned himself to an illusory fantasy of who he is.

I fear the dulling of the senses as well as that of the personality. That I won't be able to detect my apartment's musty odor as I open the door for guests, a gaunt neck sticking through the filthy collar of my undershirt, my worn witticisms and my perhaps not entirely clean cake plates, no thanks, we've actually just eaten, we do appreciate the offer (but there's hair growing from the walls).

I fear being unable to maintain the equilibrium, as I have hitherto largely succeeded in doing, of neither dismissing my bitterness nor letting myself be controlled by it—because no one reaches a certain age without accruing a degree of bitterness that one would rather not have known but which one cannot unknow again. And I tremble in fear of the resentment that would smolder within were I to convince myself that I'd all but forgotten how I was openly pissed on by my enemies and discreetly abandoned by my friends, just as, conversely, I fear becoming so possessed by anger toward the people who have wronged me that I would thereby allow them to tyrannize what precious time remains to me. At a certain point there will stand a black tower in every view, and one must neither ignore those towers—thus reducing the landscape to a simple pastoral idyll—nor become so hypnotized by them that one loses sight of the whole prospect.

I fear the erasure of secondary sexual characteristics, how softened facial features and pudgy hips make men if not womanly then at least diminished in their masculinity, while the rough skin of elder women's faces and the protruding veins of their hands diminish their womanliness, so that clothing must perform an essential role in the demarcation of sexual difference—what wonders a sharp blazer and a finely cut skirt can do to preserve our dignity as men and women, and how terribly sad it is to see an older married couple who, in their matching rain jackets and reflective athletic shoes, have totally capitulated to comfortable practicality and now resemble two liver-spotted dough balls stuffed into formless fabric sacks.

On the other hand, I also fear running into women I desired when I was young who, in defiant protest against the aging process, have now colored their hair, apparently oblivious to unsettling sight of pitch-black strands of hair drilling down into the corpse-white skin of their scalps, just as I fear that I myself will be gripped by the dotard's despair over losing his virility, which expresses itself through an obscene verbal exhibitionism for which the observer cannot reveal their distaste without being called an ageist prude. "'Don't stop! Don't stop!' she screamed while I fucked her", says the decrepit old man sitting with an IV drip, his right leg inside a monstrous gray plastic orthopedic boot.

After receiving a message this morning that an old friend had died, my first impulse was to call the poet Pia Juul so we could grieve together and reminisce about our mutual friend, but the next second it hit me that Pia isn't here anymore either. And though I do fear the possibility of slumping down in a train seat any day now, I also fear living so long that I end up alone in a rest home, staring down at an address book with all the dear names crossed out, while the most repugnant assholes are still walking around out there in high spirits, laughing in the face of God's incomprehensible plans.

And when, later in the day, I wandered over to my mother's grave in Holmen's Cemetery and remembered how the agreement between my wife and me that we would be buried together was expunged with our divorce, I felt an irrational terror at the prospect of spending eternity alone.

7

Now I hesitate at the keyboard, because, as I begin to approach the time and place where the compass needle is placed, I remember not only the intoxication of having moved to Store Kongensgade 23 but also the hopelessness, which I find almost impossible to describe, because it isn't associated with specific events that can be retrieved from my memory and shared with others, but is rather a feeling that, like my anxiety, possesses the strange duality of being at once intangible and all-pervasive. The other day I awoke to find myself completely immersed in this feeling of hopelessness in spite of having put it behind me nearly fifty years ago, but by the time I got to my desk to capture it, it had, in its spectral ineffability, already absconded. And I, who had assumed that the hopelessness of my youth would be a central theme of this essay, must now, as I attempt to put it into words, confess that the only trace that remains of it is an image of myself as a skinny, long-haired sixteen-year-old on a Sunday evening after yet another weekend visit to my old friends in Stevns, walking past the little houses and car dealerships and tacky restaurants that lined the Gammel Køge highway, hoping to catch a ride into Copenhagen, where I still didn't really know anyone. To my left, the lights of the endless apartment blocks of the city's outskirts pulsated in the September evening, and on the horizon loomed the new high rises of Brøndby Strand and the Friheden shopping center, and I have never, before or since, felt more insignificant and alien, more transparent and afraid, a random piece of rustling cellophane that might at any moment be swept up and torn apart in the nylon wind, than

I did when Bus 121 to Toftegårds Square over-took me and vanished into the darkness. That my hopelessness might have had something to do with the fact that my mother wouldn't be waiting for me at Store Kongensgade 23, because she had again been committed to a psychiatric hospital, did not occur to me.

8

And only now does it occur to me that my lifelong aversion to the provinces, while informed by the state of affairs in my downtrodden hometown fifty years ago, may also be rooted in sorrows and fears about my mother's illness that were so intense that I couldn't bear to see them when I looked inside myself, where my sorrow must have resided like a dictator. It occurs to me, too, that this sorrow became bearable (though only just) when I looked down Vestergade and took in the melancholy of its drooping little houses, the moped adorned with a fox's tail leaning up against a façade, and the defective fluorescent light flickering behind nicotine-stained nylon curtains.

And I am certainly not the only teenager from my little town who, while we were also doing our schoolwork, finding our way socially, and staring at the reliefs of the girls' sexual organs through their tight gabardine pants, had to live with their parents' misfortunes, yet it is not my overwhelming awareness of their cancer symptoms, alcoholism, or divorces, or Lars Heidemann's skeletal, sclerotic mother in her wheelchair, that first comes to mind when I consider how storm-tossed we really were, but rather the memory of the attic rooms—with their hessian wallpaper, fluttering candle lights, and jute carpeting—where we would pile onto a mattress together, seeking solace within the group, while "Bad Moon Rising" pumped through the stereo speakers and the glowing ends of our cigarettes stabbed into the dusk.

One single black-and-white image captures and concentrates for me all of the anguish every one of us must have felt, namely the image of the protagonist (almost unbearably touchingly played by a young Jesper Klein) of the film *The Ballad of Carl-Henning*, which I saw as a thirteen-year-old at Stevns Cinema in 1969: hunched over, quivering, his left hand pressing the collar of his jacket against his chest, Carl-Henning rides on his moped through a flat, misty landscape.

For reasons unknown to me, one particular place in the town continues to haunt me in hushed nightmares, namely the stretch of Algade between the town square and Egestræde, where I not infrequently dream that I'm in a state of total panic because I've realized that I can't make it back to Copenhagen. When I sought out the place a few years ago, the long-shuttered Hotel Phønix stood in an alarming state of disrepair, as if awaiting its inevitable burning. Through the gate and across the overgrown courtyard you could see the hotel's rear building, which was now so badly neglected that it seemed to be on the verge of collapsing into rubble right before your eyes, and the mere thought of crossing the courtyard, opening the door, and walking down the dank hallway to the room where we danced under the disco ball on Friday nights filled me with the same sense of disquiet that arises when one revisits reality only to have it confirmed that it is a dream.

9

While on a trip to Munich, where I was giving a reading, I stopped at an antique shop and my eyes were drawn to a magnificent Art Deco desk made of lacquered birch and inlaid with lemonwood. I fell in love with it immediately, and as my writing career had by that point reached a certain level financially, it wasn't entirely inconceivable that I might, with a bold disposition, dispatch the German beauty off to Denmark. Would it not, after all, make a worthy workplace for an acclaimed poet? My first desk, which I had in my childhood room at the house in Stevns, was a frail, scrawny thing that we ordered by mail from the Daell's Warehouse catalog, but when I moved out at seventeen, after having lived at Store Kongensgade 23 for just a year, I brought with me a dark, narrow, oaken desk that had belonged to my mother, and which was so diminutive that it could just fit beneath the window of my eight-square-meter single room with a shared kitchen on Købmagergade, where every new resident had to live until they rose within the hallway hierarchy. And when it was my turn to take over one of the larger rooms, the joyous day arrived with a relief that I couldn't comprehend until much later, as I got rid of the little inherited desk and, for the first time, acquired a piece of furniture of my very own: a bright, beautiful pinewood desk that, with a top that seems to float slightly above the legs, is a pleasure to behold and still makes me happy every day when I sit down to work. Because at the last minute I decided not to buy the Art Deco wonder and to keep my old pinewood desk, with its legs that served as a scratching post for Pjevs the Norwegian forest cat and its top on which tea and tobacco and the corrosion of daily use have all left their marks, because it suddenly hit me that it was at this desk that I'd written all of my books, from *City Slang* onwards, and just imagine if I were to get rid of it and then, sitting behind my grandiose trophy desk, discovered that I couldn't write a single word, because my books had all *grown*, so to speak, out of the pinewood desk. Which is where I am sitting right now, speculating as to what became of the little oaken desk that I first remember seeing one summer day in 1969, when I walked into my mother's room in our house in Stevns and found her sitting there just staring at the wall, which marked the beginning of seven years of madness and my adolescence.

10

My mother would later destroy her journals from 1969–76, and her memories from the period were very few in the wake of the thirty-five electroshock therapy treatments that she received in all, along with monstrous quantities of antipsychotic medicine, which included Truxal, Trilafon, Lysantin, and Sinquan—and phenobarbital and phenytoin to treat the epileptic attacks brought on by all of the psychopharmaca. However, in a document titled *Daily Life in the 1900s and Other Family Stories*, which my mother wrote in 2004 to the delight of us descendants, and in which she memorialized the lives of our family members going all the way back to 1833, the following laconic timeline emerges: in the summer of 1969, when I walked into her room and saw her sitting at the little oaken desk, my mother was suffering from extreme fatigue, and, following a thorough examination by Dr Olsen of Jernbanegade, who could not identify any physical ailments but concluded that she was depressed, she was committed to the State Psychiatric Hospital in Vordingborg, also known as Oringe, where, after five electroshock treatments, she was released, though, in her own words from the document, "unfortunately it would turn out that I was far from well". The fall of 1970 brought a commitment to Næstved Central Hospital, where they quickly decided to give her a further eight electroshock treatments, and then in August 1972, four months after the family had moved from Stevns to Store Kongensgade 23, my mother was committed to the Copenhagen Psychiatric Department (the buildings of which, at the moment of this writing, I have an unobstructed view of from my seat at the pinewood desk). She was released on 8 January 1973, but as early as 6 March of that year she found herself at Montebello in Helsingør, where she had received another fourteen electroshock treatments by the time of her release on 9 November. On 2 April 1975 my mother was committed again, this time to Sankt Hans Hospital in Roskilde, where—aside from eight weeks in the summertime—she resided for the rest of the year as she was transferred from one department to the next. In one of these departments she was treated by the psychiatrist Mogens Jacobsen, who was interested not in her half-meter-high medical records but in her, and by simply talking to her he was able to lift her out of both the depression and the medicine, so that in January 1976 she could be discharged from the psychiatric system, to which she never returned after she quickly—and permanently—stopped taking any medication. By 1 February that year she had, almost miraculously, resumed her job as a secretary. She went on to live forty good years.

11

Somewhat embarrassed upon revisiting the cocksure and not terribly incisive notes I penciled in the margins (which, in their naïve presumption of mastery, are easy to forgive), I am now looking through a book I bought the same year that my mother was discharged, namely Peter Handke's *A Sorrow Beyond Dreams*, which is about his mother's suicide. And although my mother was so unhappy that she tried to kill herself several times, she was, for the greater part of her life, so full not only of expectations but also of a satisfied contentment with existence that, in one of her many poems, she was able to write: "The world is more lovely | than any place I know | and if I go to heaven | I want to bring the world in tow". Humorous, intelligent, and sensual as my mother was, I fear that my attempt to encapsulate within these pages the place in my life where the compass needle is placed may result in my painting an overly simplistic portrait of her and her significance to me. Inspired by Orhan Pamuk's *Istanbul* and W. G. Sebald's *Austerlitz*, I at one point imagined that this book would be furnished with little black-and-white photos, but the discord between two of these pictures would, in its muted power, have reduced her to a victim—of both depression and psychiatry. The first picture comes with the caption: "Hanne and Peter. Kalundborg, 1944", and it shows my mother as a lanky thirteen-year-old who, with bright curls, a knitted sweater, a checkered dress, and woolen knee socks pulled up her pipe cleaner-thin legs, looks down tenderly at the turtle that she is cradling in her hands. I tracked down the other one by way of Morten Kirckhoff and Jan Elhøj's book *Abandoned*, which, among its pictures of abandoned places around the world, includes a selection of seven photographs of Oringe, the State Psychiatric Hospital in Vordingborg. At my request, Kirckhoff was kind enough to send me the whole series—and there it was, the photograph of a transportable electroshock apparatus. Out from a slightly rusty cabinet, which is coated in the cream-colored enamel so popular on kitchen appliances these days for a *hyggelig* retro look, there slither two black cables with electrodes to be affixed at the temples, along with a button for regulating the strength of the current and an inexplicable dial resembling that of a rotary phone. How strange it is to consider the picture of this primitive device, which could very well have been the same one that was used, when she was a grown woman, to send electricity through the brain of the bright-haired girl holding Peter the turtle in her hands in the other photograph.

12

Only once in the seven years during which my mother was committed do I remember visiting her in the hospital, because, though my father visited her every weekend when his work at the bank was finished, she didn't want me or my two younger brothers to come. I think that, on top of the depression, she was so full of shame at having been absent as a mother that it was too painful for her to see us, and, though she never spoke of it, I know from her family chronicle that she suffered for the rest of her life from guilt over not being there for us boys, who were thirteen, nine, and six years old when her illness began in 1969. But one day in 1973 she suddenly insisted that I visit her at Rigshospitalet's locked ward, and the sight of her, frightfully thin, dressed in an unwashed, pale red hospital nightgown, laughing excessively as her eyes shone unnaturally, will always live within me like a phantom. For after a series of electroshock treatments she was far from cured and seemed acutely manic instead.

It happened that a girl my own age, with whom I had never exchanged a word but had admired at a distance at the Thomas P. Hejle Youth Center on Nørrevold, was also visiting a patient, perhaps *her* mother. A friend and I called her The Bundled One, because at the youth center she always sat, in a manner typical of the time, leaned against a wall with her legs pulled up under herself and a giant sweater wrapped over her knees. She was immoderately pretty, with long, dark hair and marble-white skin decked with freckles, and when one of the female patients, dressed like the rest of them in a worn-out hospital gown, asked me to bring a plate of chocolates around to everyone in the room, I felt robbed of my dignity and completely castrated when I came to The Bundled One and dutifully extended the plate to her.

The mania left my mother just as quickly as it had come, because it was just as artificial as everything else they had plied her with in the psychiatric ward. She then became depressed again, and a professor told my father that he should focus on his sons, the implication being: because your wife isn't going to get better again. It is a remark that my father has often quoted with great bitterness toward the authority from which the judgment was issued, and which would later prove to be wrong, as my mother did in fact get better again three years later (thanks in large part to my father's love and support, the constancy of which not every man in his best years could have sustained). By a strange coincidence, it turned out that this very psychiatrist had a private clinic in the same building where my parents bought an apartment twenty years later, and though one could not have expected him to remember, after all those years, every one of his many prior patients, it would still have been a decent gesture for him to acknowledge someone he passed each day on the stairs.

And yet he is meant to be a wonderful person, at least according to what I hear from an old friend who is a patient of his. Beautiful as Nico when she was young, hysterically funny, and so intelligent that in spite of her working-class background she was the only one of us to finish her university education, she has for many years now lived her nightshade existence as a premature pensioner, strangely dazed and swollen from all the tricyclic remedies that her psychiatrist deems far more effective than those of the present day.

13

"Should the choirs of romance | Thus rise up to your lips | Exclude, if you commence | The real in its vile shapes"[1]. These lines of Mallarmé were written on a little piece of paper that I kept pinned to the wall of my dorm room. Their arrogance of course appealed to my youthful presumptuousness, but I also think that, as well as offering a warning against the cultivation of a realism that threatens to undermine the conception of poetry as an autonomous universe, they served as a personal protest against an existence that was so colored by my mother's depression—like a glass of water in which a single drop of red has dissolved—that, if I was to have a chance at becoming even somewhat grown-up, reality was going to have to remain a silence within the text right up until this autumn, forty-five years later, now that I have begun writing this book.

When I wrote previously about this essential period of my life—first and foremost in the personal essay "The Road Between Two Schools", which I wrote thirty-one years ago—I permitted myself to mention only that my mother was "sick and hospitalized for many years", without delving further into the nature of her illness ("he keeps his pain at an arm's length", as Ulrik Høy put it in his review). This was principally out of consideration for my mother, who wouldn't even speak of her gloomy years; if you so much as mentioned them then her eyes would go vacant like two little buttons, and she truly did not want the not inconsiderable collection of friends she had subsequently made through her workplaces or her winter swimming, and with whom she had a good time, to see her through the lens of that knowledge. But now, as I sit here trying to write about it all, having thought it would flow freely after my mother's death, I sense in the keys a resistance that can only come from myself.

And it is only because it is autumn, nearly winter, that I can summon the courage to keep writing, because, for reasons that I believe also have something to do with Store Kongensgade 23, autumn is *my* season, when I always feel good, even though plenty of things could, perhaps, be better. When the light dwindles to a gray fissure in the day and the big, restless foliage of the trees swoons to the ground and crunches beneath your shoes while the black skeletons of the tree trunks remain standing like inscrutable signs, and the outer world mercifully relieves us of having to bear, alone within ourselves, all that deteriorates, dies, and disappears. From the harsh light of the supermarkets we step out into the afternoon's penultimate hour, when the swarms of jackdaws gather in the trees, soon to become one with the darkness that obscures us too and circumscribes the worries of the day.

As I look back at the dates of events that transpired in the autumn of 1972, I think I know why this season, when everything ignites and dies out at once, has come to mean so much to me. It was late summer when my family moved to Copenhagen, and the first two months were very hard for me, as I hadn't found my place among my new classmates at Sølvgade School and I still missed life with my friends in Stevns, whom I now saw only on weekends, and with whom I had less in common on each visit, because, after all, we were living in separate worlds.

But when I think about my life during that autumn, the image of the weary hitchhiker on the

Gammel Køge highway is gradually supplanted by that of a young man discovering the immense city, and the loneliness fades imperceptibly into a relief at being alone and free from the gazes that pricked my neck as I walked the streets of my provincial town, which all ended in the same windswept square. And it's precisely because I came from elsewhere that Copenhagen was no mundane fact of life for me but an exotic beauty that I approached with equal shares of fear, infatuation, and intense, wide-eyed reverie about the wonders that would meet me here, where anything was possible and even the most quotidian phenomena became, in the October-dark city, objects of fascination: the column of light that suddenly illuminates a staircase down the street, the elevated train at Nørrebro Station, rattling along in close proximity to the kitchen windows where people wash their dishes, clandestine silhouettes in an archway, the twilit courtyards like nested boxes, October, when the wonderful clarity of all the white streetlamps culminates. While Store Kongensgade itself was a riot of traffic and bright storefronts, its intensity accentuated by its (for a main thoroughfare) quite narrow width, a monumental modernistic silence hung over the streets leading towards Sølvgade School, because large parts of Adelgade, Borgergade, and Sølvgade had been demolished at the beginning of the 1950s to make way for new building projects, which, just as they did back then, still stand in the same form as when they were erected, meaning that I only need to take a seven-minute bicycle ride from my current residence to be, strangely and miraculously, fifty years back in time. And especially on autumn days like today, when the streets are as deserted as they were in the '70s and all of the windows in the neighborhood's architectural crown jewel, Dronningegården, shine in the mist, I can feel how my happiness about my new life and my despair about my mother (who would be committed again by December, this time to the municipal psychiatric ward) were braided together so tightly that they became one and the same feeling.

14

It is with gratitude that I consider how, following her seven years in the psychiatric system, my mother got to have forty-two rich years before, at the age of eighty-seven, the same sickness that had decimated the lives of her mother, brother, and uncle when they were only in their fifties caught up with her as well. Despite her resolute attempt at rehabilitation after a series of violent attacks from an unknown cause, she had to forfeit her dream of, as she put it, "dipping her toes in the Øresund" again, for when she suddenly couldn't lift her head at the Norgesminde rehabilitation center, we had to concede the likelihood of Parkinson's, though no one in that strange institution, where not a single doctor is employed, had given any thought, much less reacted, to the fact that her head was hanging low on her chest and couldn't be lifted.

One day she asked my father to bring her all the poems she had written over her lifetime, and when I saw the two binders lying on the windowsill of her little room in the nursing home, it was clear to me that, if I were to avoid reproaching myself for the rest of my life, I would have to bring myself to read them all and tell her what I thought, because, in contrast to my brother Morten, who has set some of them to music, I had never really read or commented upon her poems, whereas my own had received the utmost attention, not least from her. Why had it always been so hard for me to read these poems, which I knew only in fragments? Because I was so afraid of this intimacy with my mother, to whom I was already very close, that a certain (if only inner) distance was necessary. I especially feared the poems in which she described living with depression, how it was like being buried alive, and how she was only able to hold out against death because of the love for and from my father; both things, the love as well as the suffering, were too much for me, something I ought not bear witness to. All the same, there had always been a special transmission between my mother and me, perhaps because I was not her first born but her first surviving child, after my parents' first son died in infancy.

So, while I never knew what it was that my mother was so sad about, I have, like a sonar in an underwater abyss, sensed her misery ever since I was a child, though I myself, even on the worst days, have always been too curious about tomorrow to entertain suicidal thoughts, and as I now approach old-age, in spite of my fears about the coming years, I am deeply happy to lead an existence in which most of my sorrows can be treated with such modest drugs as fine-leaf Ceylon tea from the Østerlandsk Tea Shop and strong Virginia tobacco of the Capstan Blue brand.

Reacting to my essay on reading, "Disciplined Delinquency", the journalist Rikke Viemose grumbled in *Politiken* that, out of the thirty-four books I discussed, only two were written by women. This sort of stocktaking had never occurred to me, but with a quick glance at my bookcase I can affirm that she's onto something: can it be that I prefer reading books written by men? There were several books on my family's shelves over which there seemed to reside a sort of gloom because, from what I gleaned from my parents' conversations, they were about unhappy women: among them Birgit Tengroth's *Give Me My Life Back* and, not least, Karen Stampe Bendix's *From the Thicket of My Life*, which, with its title's associations with Jesus's crown of thorns, confirmed a relationship between women, suffering, and idealization that probably already existed in my consciousness—because when our family conversations shifted to the causes of my mother's illness we would often refer to her exceptional sensitivity, for which we all loved her, thereby drawing such a firm equivalence between female suffering and female exaltation that I have anxiously seen the bones before the flesh[2] of most of the women I've fallen in love with (and whom I immediately feared would die). When I, as an adult, saw the title of Jytte Villadsen's book *Depression, Thy Name is Woman*, the words spontaneously swapped places to: Woman, Thy Name is Depression.

15

But when I walked through the door of my classroom at Sølvgade School for the first time and laid eyes on Jane, it was decidedly the flesh that I saw before the bones. Whereas the girls in Stevns had prim names like Henriette, Liselotte, and Susanne, in my new neighborhood—at that time still populated by the working classes—they were endowed with bold and snappy English names like Mercy, Kate,—and Jane, the loveliest of them all, impossible to take your eyes off, blonde and beaming like a thousand-watt bulb, with a big smile full of a teasing awareness of her radiance, which threw both the boys and the male teachers into a state of perplexity when she asked for a light, standing much too close. One evening, when I worked up the courage to call her, it turned out that I had interrupted her bath: "I'm all dripping wet", she said, causing my nightly dreams to flow over.

She was a good girl, clever and diligent at school, and in her free time she worked at the Parisian Konditori on Østerbrogade. But she was also a wild one at the Corner Discotheque on Sølvtorvet or on an acid trip in the Deer Park outside Copenhagen with Affe-Morten, Selleri, Mik-Mak, and Komet. Her family had been relocated in a slum clearance from an inner-courtyard apartment on Krystalgade, and now they lived in a high-rise with a name that couldn't be more fitting: Dronningegården[3], which, with all its shining windows and its sharp, Gothic-inspired gables, truly towered into the heavens. High-rises! Courtyards! And all the little downy hairs on Jane's thighs. And the cassette tape with "Starman" on it, which we listened to again and again.

These phenomena surreptitiously strung themselves into a chain of meaning upon which Jane's telephone number (Minerva-1936) and the rain-wet streets and her glistening sex and the days to come traded places and coalesced and became indistinguishable. How good she smelled as we lay on my bed facing the courtyard of Store Kongensgade 23, where she gave me a butterfly kiss with her eyelashes, and when, on a school trip to an even bigger city, namely London, we slipped under Marble Arch and kissed one another as the traffic swirled around us, my love for Jane coalesced with my love for a city so vast it would never end.

Most of the music that is capable of conjuring the feeling of the early '70s for me is hardly sophisticated or "progressive", as the hippy magazine *Superlove* would have had it, but considerably more poppy and catchy. It snuck into my ears from open windows and transistor radios, or through the walls of my bedroom from the bathroom, where my little brother Claus used to lie with a drink balanced on the edge of the tub while—with the door open to his own room, where "Wig-Wam Bam" and "Telegram Sam" would be thundering from the speakers—he floated in the pop soup and waited to put on his gold shirt and go out to a party. When male writers return again and again to the time of their adolescence, it is surely owing, like pop music's obsession with teenage love, to the revelation that is the first real encounter with a woman who is not one's mother. For Jane was simply happy, and, probably not unrelated to her background in Copenhagen's working class, she had a generous and uncomplicated sexuality that she offered with a laugh, without you having to wake up the next day feeling guilty about the pleasure. Nor did you become alloyed with a womanly darkness, or have to sign yourself over to one of those anxious romances from which you cannot extricate yourself, the two parties gradually winding into an indivisible thread of unspoken ambivalences. We would soon go our own ways and grow up in our own places, she in the Caribbean and I in the Copenhagen that I got to know alongside Jane, whom I think of without sentimentality but always with happiness, for she was, as Alex Michaelides writes, my "invitation to life".

16

I took the two binders of my mother's poems home and read them very slowly in the wicker chair in my little study. She had removed most of the poems that she wrote during her hospitalization—and she wrote every day—but, as I suspected and feared, a handful of the others dealt with her depression, and were constructed around the opposition between the darkness, which was her, and my father: the sun that kept her alive, though she wished herself dead.

But when I brought the poems back to her, it wasn't nearly as difficult as I had imagined it would be to sit there in her room at Norgesminde and talk about the texts, which were about plenty else besides hopeless despondency: about the seasons and silence, about the neighbor's daughter with the dark bangs, about the pleasures of red wine and memories of the streets where she'd once lived, and there was also a long series of comic nonsense poems inspired by the generation of lyricists my mother grew up with, which were executed with a finely honed linguistic craft. "The first and last lines are good, but I'm not happy with the second and third strophes, what do you think?" she would ask me, and then we would assess the advantages and disadvantages of various solutions with the unsentimental ease that now characterized our time together, which was the last thing I expected of a situation that I had assumed would summon up all manner of unbearable feelings, because my mother, after a brief and intense illness, was now paralyzed and in pain, her head stuck way down on her chest like some outlandish shellfish.

In a photo taken a few years before her Parkinson's broke out, she is wearing a very pretty red dress and a, for her, typical expression of shyness at being photographed. Had I known of the frightful condition that awaited her back when the photograph was taken, I wouldn't have thought it possible for me to be around her without seeing it all as a gruesome repetition of the suffering she had endured throughout my adolescence. Had I—through all the years that I'd feared getting too close—had an overactive imagination that was more about myself than it was about her, or had the relationship between this elderly lady and her now sixty-year-old son simply become something else? In any case, I have happy memories of those days at the facility, where we, connected without merging completely, left our inner worlds in peace and spoke mostly of practical and necessary matters: Would I buy a bouquet of flowers for Ruth for her birthday? What equipment would have to be installed before she could move back home with my father, and when might she next be granted a bath? Could I get some beer and Sprite for her room's shoddy refrigerator and bring her novels by Amos Oz, Harper Lee, and Knut Hamsun? When I saw her sitting crumpled in her wheelchair and—despite the way that Parkinson's made her slur her words, which she had to search for ever more frequently—talking excitedly about what she'd been reading, I had to ponder once again the paradoxical fate of humanity: to be furnished with a spirit that can freely roam all time and space but is chained all the while to a piece of flesh over which we are largely powerless.

I visited her every other day, and in addition to books I would bring along little things that I thought might cheer her up in the halfworld of the rehabilitation center: a small transistor radio painted her favorite shade of red, a compact mirror, an ivory comb in a leather case from Taylor of Old Bond Street, which her delicate fingers fondled affectionately. For she had always loved nice things, and keeping herself well-dressed, tidy, and beautified, with freshly painted nails and gold jewelry glittering here and there, was a necessity she refused to dispense with on account of her present diminishment—much to the contrary. So when's the hair stylist coming by?

One day, after I had closed my mother's door behind me and, a little crestfallen, started home, I passed through the common room, where my eyes landed on a cart equipped with a sign that pithily expressed the unavoidable *tristesse* of the indispensable welfare state: "Each registered resident is allocated one piece of bread/cake".

17

It's hardly surprising that one of my favorite childhood pastimes was to 'play office', because, just as my parents used to cycle off to work every morning, my father to the bank and my mother to one of the offices where she was a secretary, my grandmother was the bookkeeper at the family printing press in Kalundborg, where Aunt Inger was employed at the courthouse and Uncle Ove at an insurance company.

And secretarial work was, for my mother, a true pleasure to which she devoted herself with the duality of mirth and seriousness that is the premise of every good game. As a newly hired secretary at a messy law office, she would diligently organize and catalog all the papers, cases, and addendums into a comprehensible system of journals, binders, and cabinets, while pencils, stamps, and envelopes were also assigned their logical places. Alongside the joys of reading literature, listening to folk ballads and songs, participating in spirited debates, and swimming in the sea, office work was a lifelong source of happiness for her, beginning when she was a teenager working at the post office in Kalundborg, and then when she was employed as a 'copygirl' at *Stiftstidende*'s Copenhagen office on Laksegade, after which, on the other side of those seven years of illness, she resumed her office work, first at a pair of law offices, and then at the Technicians' Union and the Engineers' Association: if she got bored or if she wasn't valued then she would quit and quickly find a new office to straighten out.

Though it isn't uncommon for a bourgeois man to marry a working-class woman, the case of my parents was the inverse. Whereas my paternal grandmother was a cleaning lady and my grandfather a factory worker (who died at sixty of a lung cancer that can likely be attributed to the toxic powder that the workers at the sulfuric acid plant in Kalundborg shoveled straight off of the floor without any kind of protection), my mother's grandfather, Albert Vejlø, started out as an editor at the Kalundborg newspaper before becoming the proprietor of Vejlø's Printing Press on Kordilgade, while also serving a brief stint as a conservative parliamentarian. He lived in an imposing villa that, in his provincial bourgeois majesty, he built up on a hilltop overlooking the whole town. And my maternal grandmother's siblings carried on their bourgeois heritage: there was Karen, who earned a master's degree in political science, immigrated to the United States, and was employed in the Department of Agriculture during Roosevelt's final New Deal administration, Børge, who was an engineer who worked with Kampsax in Persia to build the Trans-Iranian Railway and would later live in the small yet grand Hercules Pavilion in the King's Garden, and Volmer, who took over the printing press and, in his lovely modern villa overlooking the water on Gisselørevej, lived the good life with Aunt Kiss and their four fashionable, intelligent children, who to my ten-years-younger child-eyes exuded a Kennedyesque glamour as they leaned their long, suntanned bodies into the wind in their optimist sailboats out on the Kalundborg Fjord.

If my maternal grandmother's life took on a more modest, one might even say poorer, trajectory, it is first because (like her sister Bitten) she received no education apart from what she learned by helping her father in the office of the printing press, and secondly because she, herself a stunning beauty, married the handsome and charismatic young journalist Henning, who was easy to fall in love with but who, with his histrionic temperament, was far from being a responsible spouse to my grandmother, regardless of how many love poems he wrote her—and he was just as far from being a reliable father to their children, my mother and her two brothers. On the countless occasions that I've speculated about the possible causes of my mother's depression, my thoughts have always returned to my grandfather, or rather: to my mother's life with *her* downtrodden mother and this fascinating, erratic father figure, from whom I've been told that I inherited the habit of restlessly pacing the floor but whom I never met, as he died of a brain infection in a rented room in Copenhagen in April 1945 (when my mother was thirteen years old), separated for the third time from my grandmother, who in her succeeding forty-nine years as a widow kept Henning's portrait hanging over her bed, which may have been the one place in this world where she could truly make contact with that man, who, when he saw himself in the mirror each morning, would proclaim: "I'm handsome as Adonis!"

Henning's instability extended into the life of the family; their address changed fourteen times in as many years, because, for unknown reasons, his tenures as a journalist at, for example, *Østsjællands Folkeblad*, *Frederiksborg Amts Avis*, *Børsen*, and *Ringkøbing Amts Avis* were always short-lived. In the places where he couldn't bring his wife and children, he lived in temporary lodgings, while my grandmother had to scrape by with the children and endure such humiliations as the repossession of her dining room furniture by the bailiff for unpaid hotel and restaurant bills. Whether my grandfather was fired or quit—and why—we don't know, but my mother's family chronicle, which I have to thank for all of this factual documentation, reports that he was frequently hospitalized and operated upon because of head pains relating to a receding mandible and sinus infections until, as his doctors had predicted, he got his fatal brain infection, which would've been knocked out with penicillin a few years later.

"If you want to talk to Volmer then you'll have to come right away", Aunt Kiss told me, "because he won't live much longer". So I took the train to Kalundborg to hear Uncle Volle tell me of his youthful admiration for the thirteen-years-older Henning and (previously unbeknownst to me) his disappointment and anger at the man's recklessness. I'll never forget the atmosphere of that late winter day in 1997, a steel-gray storm ripping at the waves on the fjord, as Volmer, who had a hospital bed installed in the villa on Gisselørevej, lay in the dusky living room and, looking out at the restless waters, concluded his account with the proclamation: "Your grandfather was a psychopath". This was all the more shocking because I had never before heard Volmer, the soul of kindness and discretion, speak critically of anyone. When I discussed the matter several years later with one of Aunt Kiss and Volmer's sons, who had become a doctor, he suddenly grew quiet, and then he said that, knowing what we know of Henning's erratic mind, his unmoored existence, and his constant physical afflictions, one might, perhaps, draw the conclusion that he was syphilitic. A theory that I never shared with my mother, who'd had more than enough to speculate about in her life.

When my grandfather died, it turned out that—irresponsible to the last (or was the brain infection to blame?)—he had not paid the final premium of his life insurance, which was thereby nullified. The only supplement that my grandmother, now alone with three children, had to her modest salary from the printing press was 27 kroner and 79 øre per month from the Danish Journalists' Guild, plus 100 kroner at Christmastime, for which she wrote a thank you letter every year.

Among her modest confirmation gifts, my mother remembered in particular a flounder skin handbag that quickly became cracked, and it was only as an adult that I grasped how poor my grandmother really was, because as a child I had seen her as something of a cosmopolitan lady. Though she didn't have the means to take over the family villa on the hilltop after her parents died and lived instead in a tiny house on the shabby side of town, alongside communists and with the stench of the slaughterhouse hanging in the air, she maintained her bourgeois Mrs Vejlø-dignity, gracious and courteous towards all the shopkeepers and uncommonly elegant in the pretty dresses that her sister Karen sent from Washington. When I received the Aarestrup Medal in 1991, my eighty-six-year-old grandmother gave me a very little book, only slightly larger than a matchbox, which contained a selection of Emil Aarestrup's *Love Poems*. It had been a gift to her from Henning.

18

Who my grandfather was, what my mother was really sad about, what Mogens Jacobsen said to her, why the friends of my parents' youth, who I found so charming, almost all suddenly disappeared when my mother got sick, what became of them, and what, other than a nameless angst, actually happened to me during my adolescence, I don't know. Whenever I pass by the apartment in Store Kongensgade 23 it is always, strangely enough, empty, so please forgive the fact that you are sitting with a book that is, correspondingly, about all the things the author doesn't know. On the other hand: The things I know, I don't need to write about, because I already know them.

One day in my mid-twenties, in an attempt to find out something that I didn't know, I went to see another psychoanalyst, and this time it turned out to be the right one. After a consultation with a female psychiatrist I walked crestfallen through the city, absolutely certain that this otherwise very lively and appealing person would never be able to help me. When I passed by a telephone booth, I went in, opened the phone book to the yellow pages, and called the secretary of the Danish Psychoanalytic Society, John Vigter, who suggested that we have a few preliminary conversations so that both parties could determine whether this was the right way forward.

My path to psychoanalysis started with a renunciation of psychiatry that was based on its treatment of my mother and was then furthered by the so-called antipsychiatry movement, which, in the spirit of the times, perceived the established treatments as a component in the suppression of the individual by 'society'. Ronald D.

Laing's books, published in lovely slim editions by Bibliotek Rhodos, still sit on my shelf, but as brilliant as these texts are in many respects, the prospect of a treatment based on their precepts was vague. And though the movement's frenzied, ideological nature was perhaps persuasive to me as a young man, it was not sufficient sustenance to me as a slightly older one, one who had begun studying at the Institute for Comparative Literature, where the generation of '68 introduced me to psychoanalysis, whose insistence that what a person says or writes actually *means* something and is a key to understanding seemed more convincing than psychiatry's conception of the psyche as the product of biochemical processes.

I consider those rebellious students' resumption of the serious study of Freud, following decades of neglect by people who only knew his work from primitive surveys and whose pompous verdict was that "science left that stuff behind a long time ago", to be one of that generation's greatest accomplishments, and it saddens me that psychoanalysis has been marginalized in the universities' psychology departments, even as it flourishes in a less-than-pure form, with an accompanying (and unfortunately understandable) loss of dignity, on the yoga mats of so many homespun psychotherapeutic offices, where I personally would no sooner seek help than in a psychiatric hospital.

And just as the generation of '68 have been like my intellectual big brothers and sisters—from whom I've learned such a great deal and whose views I still share to a large extent, no matter how much we may sometimes have disagreed during our valuable and always delightful conversations—so also was Vigter, who was born in

1928, a *grand old man* for those of the '68-ers who went on to study and practice psychoanalysis.

As soon as I stepped into Vigter's big, pretty, corner office overlooking the park around Montebello in Helsingør, where he was the superintendent, I knew I had come to the right place, and in the years that followed I would take my place in that chair every week and talk about my daily life, about my family and my past, about my thoughts, desires, and bad dreams, while he interjected only occasionally with a comment or a tentative interpretation that was always held at a distance and never absolute. In the beginning I was disappointed, in my childish eagerness, not to be approved as a classic analysand (who lies on the sofa four times a week), but a less intensive treatment soon proved to be the right decision. Instead of surrendering completely to my inner world, I could sit face to face with the analyst as he held my gaze calmingly and supported me during the temporary retreats that took place when the material became too overwhelming—because it goes without saying that the path to liberating awareness was sometimes so upsetting that I didn't want to say one word more.

If you're expecting these years to be recounted as a dramatic case story in which, at a certain point, the penetrating analyst will assemble enough evidence to strike upon a specific event or encapsulate the problem in a single eye-opening assessment, then I will have to disappoint, because I can only describe what happened as a process wherein one person's ineffable angst, in the encounter with another's interpretations, gaze, and silence, gradually transformed into language and slowly lost ground—not to a point at which I could be deemed 'well' by some normative standard, but to the extent that I could now live my life. For this to work, it is necessary that the two parties feel elementally compatible, and that the patient's subjective interest in gaining awareness is met by the analyst's interest in gathering knowledge, just as the analysand must have faith in the analyst's ability to a degree that, in the beginning, approaches idealization, which the analyst, in turn, must not crave.

And Vigter clearly didn't, for he rested easily within himself. He was friendly, humorous, and intelligent, both highly observant and gently reserved, and always dressed in a jacket and tie—attesting to the formal rather than personal character of our relationship. He mastered the delicate balance of inhabiting another person's most intimate world while also maintaining a comfortable distance, which is the precondition for both parties being at ease in the situation and coming to awareness within that rarified, consciously artificial space. And he knew how to accommodate an acute need for acknowledgment, encouragement, and reassurance without letting himself be manipulative or neglecting, when necessary, to assume a role that did not correspond with my wishes, and perhaps directly opposed or pulled the rug out from under them.

Naturally, the impetus to begin psychoanalysis always stems from something being wrong, but unless the longing for a less vexed existence is truly oppressive, very few people are likely to tolerate the discomfort that is a necessary aspect of the treatment. Something surprising happened toward the end of my years with Vigter, which is that our focus shifted imperceptibly from the question of why I was feeling so bad to the inverse question of why I was fundamentally doing so well, and of why, in spite of everything, I looked forward each day to the next. And while there was no doubt that my mother's illness played a major role in the angst that arose during my adolescence, right when my boyhood self's natural separation from his mother should've been picking up steam but was instead restrained out of concern for her, it was equally clear that I had this very same mother's love—along with my father's dependability—to thank for the fact that, even on my worst days, I am also always doing all right.

19

From Store Kongensgade 23 I remember the oppressive atmosphere that quickly set in each time my mother was discharged after being deemed healthy once again, which was getting harder and harder to swallow. I remember the mute shame of watching how she fought each time to live up to that illusion, even as she grew more transparent with every passing day, until finally she fell apart again and had to be committed anew.

"Suicide as language", I jotted down at the age of twenty on page 68 of *A Sorrow Beyond Dreams*, and in spite of my youthful naïvete I was on the right track, for I wish that my mother had had the same opportunity that I later had to understand, step by linguistic step, the reasons for her suffering, and that she hadn't been subjected to seven years of violent and ineffectual psychiatry before she happened to meet a doctor who attempted to grasp what she said to him. Naturally, when they told her that "mental illness is like a broken bone, nothing to be ashamed of", they did so with the best of intentions, namely to remove the shame of being in the locked ward. But, at the same time, the expression's analogy between the psychic and the somatic is telling of a psychiatry that understands states of mind to be biologically determined. Within this framework, what a patient says can't possibly lead to an understanding of the illness, because it is, in itself, of no importance—merely a product of the true, biochemical cause. But the fact that the brain is the seat of consciousness does not mean that soma and psyche, body and soul, are the same, and I am amazed at how psychiatric practitioners, with their strange lack of intellectual curiosity, can listen to the characteristic speech of the depressed or psychotic without it occurring to them that something so filled with meaning cannot just be a random symptom, but must instead disclose something essential about the illness itself.

Don't get me wrong: I'm not on a moralistic crusade for natural purity, and I certainly believe that psychopharmaca can be necessary in acute situations to prevent suicide or ameliorate dangerous aggressions and unbearable angst. What I'm calling into question is something far more fundamental than the obvious pragmatic uses of these drugs—namely the idea that they are capable of healing the root cause of a mental illness. In her book *The Myth of the Chemical Cure*, Joanna Moncrieff distinguishes between two conceptions of psychopharmaca: "the disease-centred" and "the drug-centred model of drug action". While the latter is solely concerned with drugs' effects on the psyche, "the disease-centred model" proposes that they can, in a targeted fashion, correct the chemical imbalance presumed to be the cause of the illness, and therefore that the medicine not only treats symptoms but actually heals.

In Raban Rosenberg's article "Psychopharmalogical Developments, 1950-1970", one reads that: "It would later be found that the anti-depressive effects of both imipramine and the subsequently developed drugs within the so-called tricyclic class of antidepressants is due to their effect on signal transmission between brain cells... This research corroborated one of early pharmacology's theoretical flagships: that the disturbance of signal transmission between brain cells is the central disorder not only in schizophrenia, but also in the great classic illness itself, manic-depressive psychosis".

This is a conclusion arrived at in reverse—moving from effect to cause: because these drugs affect signal transmission between brain cells, their anti-depressive effect must be due to the fact that depression is caused by a dysfunction of said signal transmission. I have furthermore never seen a convincing argument for the connection between a biological defect and a specific psychological symptom—such as my mother's debilitating self-criticism and feelings of worthlessness. While it may reasonably be asserted that a specific drug's effect on signal transmission between brain cells has an anti-depressive effect, the argumentation for the opposite line of reasoning (between a failure of signal transmission and the patient's symptoms) consists, as far as I can see, of so many missing links that it is difficult to accept. What *is* self-evident, however, is that, far from addressing a discrete biological process, these drugs immerse the entire consciousness in a chemical soup, which in my mother's case transformed her into a pitiful sleepwalker and hindered an intelligent woman from reflecting on what was happening inside her.

A few years ago, when I suggested to a publishing house—one I considered to be classically humanist, in the term's academic rather than its sentimental sense—that they translate and publish Moncrieff's book, I was resolutely rejected, and I'm aware that I am embarking into particularly sensitive territory here. The critique of these treatments often arouses an understandable anger, both among the doctors who, with scanty resources and in far from ideal working conditions, are truly doing their best, and among the patients who've had good experiences with psychiatry. But that doesn't invalidate my own anger or my personal experiences, which I've had more than four decades to ponder, and which, after my mother's death, I now feel free and justified, and perhaps even obligated, to share, for just as autumn is *my* season, this is my book, and as a counterweight to Mallarmé's admonition against allowing poetry to be submissive to reality, I will include here one of Paul Éluard's poems, which reads in its entirety: "I say what I see | what I know | what is true".

20

I stuffed myself with great quantities of horror films during my first years as a Copenhagener, and there was one film in particular that I watched again and again, namely William Friedkin's *The Exorcist,* released in 1973. If teenagers have a large appetite for the cinematic terrors that we adults can't bear—"because age has made us innocent", as the poet Henrik Nordbrandt writes—it is likely because they unleash a joyous catharsis of all the pent-up fears that we carry during those years, in both inner and outer worlds that we don't have much control over.

And I have no doubt that it was because of a (as I remember it, unconscious) feeling of powerlessness at not being able to help my mother that I was affected not least by the film's parallel storyline about the young priest haunted by feelings of guilt because he can't afford a private nursing home for his senile mother, who must be admitted to a dilapidated public institution alongside insane women who, plaintive and pleading, accost him and grasp at him when he comes to visit. This scene seemed much more powerful to me than the grotesque extremes for which the film is infamous. Enamored as I was with *The Exorcist,* there was one point at which I would always shut my eyes (and which I actually didn't really see until a few years ago, when I finally wrote an essay about the work), namely the scene where the possessed girl, affixed to big noisy machines, undergoes several painful medical procedures, the names and purposes of which I didn't know but doubtless associated with the electroshock my mother was receiving while I sat in the theater-dark.

Instead of counting ECT, *electroconvulsive therapy*, as a fortunate modern scientific breakthrough, I regard the idea of a shock cure as being far from new; it is, rather, an age-old psychiatric dream of taking a shortcut past the perplexing nature and drawn-out treatment of mental illness. In the beginning of the 1800s, doctors in the Berlin asylum carried out shock treatment with the help of a so-called centrifuge, which patients were strapped into and then, to their distress, whirled around, just as, even longer ago, the insane were marched out onto a bridge where a trap door would spring open, plunging the patient into an ice cold lake, and with this shock they were believed to be healed. From 1933 until the early '50s, cardiazol shock therapy and insulin coma therapy were considered to be nothing less than miracles (whose time, like that of all miracles, ended suddenly). An injection of cardiazol would provoke an epileptic seizure, which was seen as curative because, according to an article by Jesper Vaczy Kragh in the book *Psychiatry's History in Denmark*, there was thought to be a "biological antagonism between epilepsy and schizophrenia" (because rates of schizophrenia were observed to be lower among epileptics). Manfred Sakel, the originator of insulin coma therapy, meanwhile believed that "insulin blocked the most active brain cells—deemed to be the root cause of the psychosis—while simultaneously strengthening the 'normal pathways'", which may sound familiar, as it mirrors today's equally opaque belief that electroshock stimulates the formation of new brain cells, which depression is presumed to inhibit.

That some patients experience undeniable—if only temporary—relief from depression following electroshock is more or less a pragmatic justification for the method, and yet I remain uneasy about it for several reasons. And here I'm thinking primarily neither of injuries nor of other complications, for what bothers me most of all is that, as in the case of psychopharmaca, the focus is largely on effects rather than causes. What's more, I see no reason to explain away my spontaneous understanding of those terrifying spasms as a form of torture and punishment by saying that this reaction would be more at home in the nursery room than in the enlightened world—as long as science, which is meant to trump obscurantism with rationality, doesn't seriously deal with the content of what the patient actually says about their own troubles. For though it may be that mental illness can be defined as a dysfunction of neurotransmitters—the usual suspects—it doesn't follow that this defect is necessarily the fundamental cause of the illness.

That it is of such paramount importance for psychiatry to link the psychic to the somatic, thereby losing its way as I see it, is likely owing to the field's eternally frustrated ambition to be recognized as a real, evidence-based science and a rightful member of the medical republic, rather than tolerated as a semi-literate cousin from the countryside. Consider, for example, this excited passage from *Doctors' Weekly*, 1949 (cited in the aforementioned article), in which we read that it "is inarguable that psychiatry is at present the most expansive of the medical disciplines". It "cannot be denied", the article continues, "that clinical psychiatry has made major steps forward, grounded in clear scientific method". And "electroshock therapy—alongside insulin treatment and the prefrontal lobotomy—is our era's most significant contribution to the somatic treatment methods within psychiatry". One distinctly senses the text's delight in its coldly clinical vocabulary, which turns psychiatry away from the subjective focus of the humanistic fields and towards a harder, objective science.

My mother received a diagnosis of "endogenous depression", and this expression annoys me because, with its medical-Latinate aura of expertise, it postulates a knowledge that it doesn't have, since it just means: as we cannot see any external reasons for the illness, it must come from within (which is to say, we have no idea). The way that an old friend whom I meet on the street every now and then tells me one year that she's bipolar and the next that she's borderline and has therefore had to change her prescription is one of the many reasons why I have little faith in the capacity of these diagnoses to articulate anything meaningful. Similarly, the fact that so inconceivably many young people today are supplied with a psychiatric diagnosis, which they proceed to identify with in the belief that the magical acronym—ADD, OCD, ADHD—more or less sums up their entire person, hinders, as I see it, the individual's understanding of themself as a unique and manifold being who's also been affected by their upbringing and the broader circumstances of their life.

Far from being rational, the psychiatric world seems to be characterized by the colorful superstition that its treatments will be more scientific if they involve chemicals and machines, blood tests and graphs full of numbers. Many years ago in the Copenhagen University Library's collection on Nørre Allé, I found an article by medical director Einar Geert-Jørgensen and his colleagues at the Frederiksberg Hospital concerning their crazy experiments with LSD in the early '60s, in which, with the aid of misunderstood, banalized concepts imported from psychoanalysis, they reasoned that the supposedly curative effects of LSD hallucinations were brought about when repressed material was liberated and, with the wave of a magic wand, integrated into the patient's personality (this argument was later invalidated in many cases, and common sense tells us that it's precisely not the mentally ill, but only the exceptionally well-balanced, who can handle these powerful hallucinogens). It astounds me that they ever risked experimenting with LSD on those already fragile patients, especially as, on the one hand, they were well aware of the drug's intensity, while, on the other, they had such a vague understanding of its effects on specific symptoms that they tested it on such widely varying phenomena as anxiety, depression, impotence, schizophrenia, writer's block, and transvestism (!) with the aim of gradually homing in on the indication area—just as it astounds me how contemporary psychiatry invertedly perceives disturbances in neurotransmission to be the origin of countless different symptoms, even though each of those symptoms speaks its own language.

I am further amazed at how the same article presents the information that two suicides, four suicide attempts, and one murder took place among the patients during the experiments in a neat little graph, though these facts could easily have been expressed in text. I suspect that this peculiarity is owning to graphs having a more 'scientific' aspect than text, whose many possibilities for personal tone, ambivalence, and nuance risk eroding the semblance of objectivity.

Perhaps these sorrowful deeds also become easier to endure when, organized into a graph, they are refined into clinical observations made in service of research.

I got a further insight into the self-perception of psychiatry—or, more correctly, of the psychiatrist—when, in the international psychiatric journals that I found in the University Library, I stumbled upon advertisements for psychopharmaca, which typically showed a male psychiatrist towering in patriarchal dominion behind a heavy mahogany desk, before which a pathetic, distraught patient sits squirming. The interesting thing is that the group at which these advertisements are aimed is none other than the psychiatrists themselves, so their endorsement of a certain product's positive effects on the patient is simultaneously an advertisement for the phallic inviolability that comes with the power to prescribe it.

"We have much better options today" is the soothing refrain that has sounded every decade—from the heralding of 'holiday pills' (amphetamines) over barbiturates in the 1950s, to the benzodiazepines of the '60s, to today's SSRIs, known in Denmark as 'happy pills', the positive benefits of which are hotly debated (even as their side effects are universally acknowledged). Personally, I have a hard time seeing what progress has been made, given that electroshock is still widely administered in Denmark, experimentation with psychedelic drugs has resumed (this time it's psilocybin), and, as recently as 2012, there was a major crisis within the Capital Region's "Psychiatry of the Future" project when its illustrious pioneer, the clinical director of the Glostrup Psychiatric Center, was dismissed after the press informed us that his success rate with quick discharges—the so-called 'accelerated treatment courses' that were enthusiastically copied in many of the capital's psychiatric wards—was due to the patients being rendered utterly passive with life-threatening megadoses and dangerous combinations of medications such as Leponex, Midazolam, and Zyprexa (note that these are not the names of the drugs' active ingredients but names invented by marketing departments, which, with their fondness for the 'exotic' letters *z* and *x*, imbue these products with a certain mystic quality). When there are 690,000 people in the country currently taking psychopharmaca, which makes us one of the world's biggest consumers of this kind of medicine, there is cause to consider whether the sudden, early, 'unexplained' deaths among psychiatric patients may be associated with these drugs, many of which are known to lead to obesity, diabetes, strokes, and heart attacks.

Being a psychiatric patient has never been a cheerful affair, but, with all the radical interventions and cures that became available, including the lobotomy ('the white cut'), electroshock therapy, and treatment with hallucinogens and heavy psychopharmaca, the twentieth century seems to me like the Dark Ages of psychiatry. Pardon the expression, but it's been burning on my tongue for forty years.

21

"I remember everyone", my mother said on her deathbed, where she had suddenly begun speaking English, and I'm certain that she really did remember everyone she'd ever met, just as they never forgot her. At once serious and humorous, and always attuned to the individual sitting across from her, she would listen with intelligent empathy to everything that was said to her, whether in a private setting or a lively group. My parents always had a wide circle of friends, from back at age seventeen when they founded their "Club of Forty-Nine" along with some friends, until their later years, when I would walk into their apartment to find my mother with two or three old ladies unknown to me, all hunched over a Scrabble board like crows around a pizza box. I have not infrequently been approached after readings and lectures around the country by someone I didn't know but who had met my mother at some point—at a workplace or a *højskole*[4], or while winter swimming—and wanted to express their gratitude and respect, and to send their regards.

"The Danish Language Council, Vester Voldgade 115", it says in my mother's big, looping handwriting on the first page of my inherited copy of the *Berlingske Dictionary of Foreign Words*. The Language Council undoubtedly received many inquiries from her, because if there was one thing that interested my mother, it was language. The love of language is something she and I always shared: in a beautiful black-and-white photograph that I now have framed here in my apartment, I'm sitting in her lap and we're both looking down in concentration at an open book (which must be a picture book, since I'm just a pudgy little toddler).

While art has been my father's passion, reading and discussing literature was hers, and in her later years, when she was bound to her wheelchair and I served as her book delivery service, I had to be judicious with my selections: a new Danish novel was cast aside with the assessment that "she writes like a girl in eighth grade", while she read aloud from Elena Ferrante's *My Brilliant Friend* with delighted laughter. While my generation grew up with English, and the following ones even more so, it really was a foreign language for my parents, and for as long I can remember my mother was trying to learn it in evening classes—but she was too shy to speak it until her final days. Had they been born ten years later, I'm certain that my parents would've been academics, my father an art historian and my mother in one of the linguistic fields, but this was unthinkable for them, as there wasn't yet any public financial aid for education, and neither my mother's mother nor my father's parents were able to support grown children—quite the contrary, as my mother had to supplement my grandmother's monthly salary from the printing press, which on 1 May 1951, after fixed costs but before taxes, came to 165 kroner even. But in the end it may have been a blessing that neither my father nor my mother received a university education, for I believe that, by earning their money from other sources and devoting themselves to their interests only after working hours, they actually got the best from the worlds of art and literature, which were preserved for them in all their glory, immune to the power struggles, animosities, and more or less disappointed ambitions that easily follow when passions are professionalized. In any case, it was both a joy and an inspiration to their son to grow up in a wonderland of walls crowded with artwork and shelves full of the books that my father, with his salary as a bank assistant as collateral, purchased on credit, at first from Elling's Bookshop in Kalundborg and later from Harck Bookshop on Fiolstræde in Copenhagen, in whose yearly sales catalog I was also permitted to place my crosses.

While his love of art and interior design has always spurred my father to invest in new houses, apartments, paintings, books, and furnishings, the frugality of my mother's childhood home, combined with her inherited bourgeois self-discipline, served as a counterweight, and I remember from Stevns how she divided our household money into various envelopes, each with its own heading: *food, clothes, transportation, additional expenses.* All things considered, the substantial differences between these two people are likely a significant reason why their marriage—in spite of my mother's long periods of illness, during which, with depressive self-loathing, she tried in vain to convince him to find someone else—lasted all the way from the Club of Forty-Nine until her death in 2020. My mother: thoughtful, rational, and, despite all her understanding of others, a person who was, so to speak, turned inward, while my father, with his interest in concrete reality and his immense factual knowledge about everything from the color palette of Golden Age painters to the baking of rye bread, was turned outward, toward a world he's always felt at home in, and which, notwithstanding all the aggressive old-man illnesses he's now saddled with, he is never too tired to explore.

When I look at the photograph of my father in which, as a three-year-old in a sweater and breeches with a gleeful smile on his face, he radiates the same inner satisfaction with existence that he does this very day eighty-six years later, I envy his robustness, but when I look at the picture of young Hanne, tenderly holding a turtle in her hands, I have an urge to lift her up protectively in mine. And I remember my mother's story of how Henning told her they were going to "visit a little girl" when in truth they were on the way to a hospital where my mother was to have an operation, and I remember my father telling me how my grandmother Emilie, who went by Emily, would, when they went swimming at the beach, draw her wet little son inside her robe to warm him with her body.

22

Why all my parents' friends vanished from our lives—here one day and gone the next—I don't really know. Though it likely had something to do with my mother's illness, the beginnings of which in 1969 coincided with this great disappearing act, I am once again forced to write of something I don't know much about.

But I do remember that the atmosphere in our house in Stevns during the years leading up to the great silence was intensely lively and festive, with a big flock of friends, all in their mid-thirties, gathering almost every weekend at my parents' house, where they ate and drank, lit their cigarettes and pipes, laughed and conversed, took walks around the bog or down along the cliffside, danced to the music on our four-track Tandberg reel-to-reel tape player, or gathered around the piano and sang along as my mother played tunes from the *Fireside Book of Folk Songs*. How beautiful and fascinating they were as they arrived in the nifty little cars that the middle classes could now also afford; a black Volkswagen and a red Morris Mascot in the driveway boded well. And I admired all of them boundlessly: Max, who was a taxi driver for Codan Cars on Halmtorvet and was also studying Danish literature with the famous professor Aage Henriksen; Erik, who was a schoolteacher at the rowdy Fælledvejen School in Nørrebro (where the girls did handstands when he passed by on the stairs so that their dresses would fall down) and, with his jet-black hair and an ironic glint in his eye, was one of the coolest people I'd ever seen, a real Copenhagener; and then their pretty wives, the light-haired, Finnish Leila, and Kirsten, who looked like an Italian film star and was quick to laugh in my company. I would listen, enchanted, to Max after lunch as he leaned back his impressive bald head and tossed out labyrinthine literary ideas that no one else could really follow, while everyone, including us kids, who again didn't fully grasp what was going on (or did we?), relished the sparking atmosphere, wherein masculinity was paraded bare-chested above the lawnmower while the women relaxed in lounge chairs and rubbed their suntanned arms with Nivea cream. Best of all was when my mother ran her hand down my neck as she said goodnight: a summer night lying in bed on the first floor and listening to the far-off voices and laughter of the adults, drifting off to sleep but also right there at the big party. Which ended so suddenly.

Did they disappear like a flock of startled birds because my mother had been overcome by an impenetrable darkness, or did something happen between them to unleash a depression that was, perhaps, always latent within her? I've speculated about this a great deal, though I'm not sure I want to know the answer, which isn't to be found in her family history, where, strangely enough, none of these once so important people is mentioned with as much as a word. This omission was my mother's choice to make, and I have no right to challenge it, because just as Store Kongensgade 23 is, for me, the place where the compass needle sits (whereas for my brothers and parents it may only be one address on their path through life), it may be that these people whom I saw with the enchanted eyes of a child actually meant more to me than they did to my father and mother, whose silence about this high point in my childhood I must respect, for "one sometimes endeavors to forget the little cluster of people who shaped the beginning of one's life", as Patrick Modiano writes in *Memory Lane*.

But I can't help thinking that the friendship within this group of young grown-ups was probably a bit too intense—a few of the couples had even moved to our little village to be closer to the others (though they were all too bourgeois for true collective living), and I know from my own youth how mutual adoration within the magnetic field of a circle of friends can imperceptibly obscure boundaries in a way that only becomes apparent once it's too late. And it *was* too late: "Can you settle my bill at the grocery store?" was the last thing my father heard from Erik, who had gotten divorced from Kirsten, after which they both moved away and out of sight.

How young they all look in the old snapshots whose subjects are becoming washed out as the fading colors retreat into the paper. Only a few details about the missing can be gleaned from the internet, which ostensibly tracks the movements of every single contemporary person—but, then again, it was created long after these people's youth. So if you want to find out what happened to Max Røbel, Erik Kobbelvedt, Niels Henrik Hørlyck, and their lovely wives (who may have long since remarried and taken other last names), you'll get lost in your own Modiano novel, in which the elusive, ghostly fates you seek are circumscribed by highly concrete facts such as dates, telephone numbers, and addresses. If, for example, you search for "Erik Kobbelvedt", you're certain to find a handsome, dark-haired boy (who looks a lot like the grown man I knew) standing sixth from the left in the first row of the Skolen ved Sundet (Samosvej 50) second-grade class photo from 1947–8. And then on 1 January 1970 (the year after he moved away from Stevns) he registered as a member of the homeowners' association of Baunehøj Park, 3500 Værløse. But there the trail runs dry.

23

Yes, what becomes of us? Over the twenty-five years that I've been sitting around the table at The Danish Academy's meetings in Rungstedlund, I've noticed, as the years have gone by, that neither deceased nor retired members, whose presence and judgment meant so much only a moment ago, are mentioned with as much as a word. That these former members appear—as of the very first meeting after their departure—never to have existed is probably due neither to any aversion nor to some quality unique to this particular body, but simply to the social law that, as soon as we've stood up and started for the door, an unknown hand passes over our faces and erases them forever.

24

After her stay at the rehabilitation center and before her protracted death in the hospital, my mother lived at home with the apartment (to my father's dismay) full of outlandish machines that lifted her into and out of the bed and hauled the wheelchair up and down the stairs, while caregivers let themselves in five times a day to help her bathe, take her to the toilet, and make her bed.

When you came into the living room, she would be sitting with her back to you, her unmoving head hanging low, so that in order to greet her you had to crouch down and look up into her face, which would beam down at her guest with the most lively, clear, and—incredibly enough—humorous expression. Next to her wheelchair's permanent spot at the table she had, true to form, arranged an efficient office, complete with writing utensils, folders, and a rolling file cabinet, so that she could reach everything from the spot to which she had been fixed. When her organizational system went so far that, to the benefit of potential burglars, she collected all her user-names and passwords into a binder on whose spine she carefully wrote "Secret Codes", we couldn't help but laugh, just as she had to laugh at herself when the hallucinations induced by her Parkinson's medication convinced her that she had just returned from Switzerland, when in fact she hadn't moved a bit in months. Nailed to one place but with her big radar spinning, she would always ask elaborate questions about the people you knew and had seen recently, so when she stopped playing along in her best friends' Wordfeud game they had good cause to worry.

She was admitted to urgent care at Bispebjerg Hospital three times, each time after losing consciousness at home in the apartment. On one occasion seven or eight alarmed nurses and doctors suddenly surrounded her and rolled her off to yet another operation. During the fearful nighttime hours that followed, the whole family gathered under the grimy light fixtures in the main hall of that rickety little high-rise that every taxi driver knows as Bispebjerg Bakke 23, Hall 60. When she awoke after the operation and it was my turn to visit her in the intensive care unit, where she lay with tubes and wires and little blinking machines everywhere, I feared that the supply of oxygen to her brain might have been interrupted—and yet there seemed to be a bit more color in her cheeks. I said she was looking better than last I saw her, to which she responded: "I wish I could say the same about you", and then I knew that my mother's mind, at least, had not come to any harm.

Among hospital personnel she was known as "the lady with the black book", because no matter which department she'd been moved to, she always brought along the second volume of Lars Saabye Christensen's *Echoes of the City*, which, despite her rapidly dwindling strength, she was trying to keep on reading. But she steadily slipped into a state that tipped between unconsciousness and a strangely unreal clarity, and when I asked her how she was doing one day, she answered with a remarkable formulation: "I have a feeling that I'm doing very well", which makes a kind of sense, because all the love that she had sent out into the world was now coming back to her, as much from the close family members who were gathered around her bed day and night as from the people she had met throughout her life and who constantly shone on that far-reaching radar of hers.

She lived long enough to hold the little book of her selected poems, which my younger brother Morten had gotten printed under the title *Hanne Wrote*, in her hands with great joy and satisfaction, and though she gradually disappeared almost entirely as the days went by, she still reacted from somewhere deep within to words like "red wine" and "gold jewelry", for her sensuous delight in pleasure and beauty was so strong that on her way to heaven she took the world in tow (as Hanne wrote in one of her early poems), and though she probably didn't really register it herself, I'll never forget the moment when my ex-wife, Nanette, and my stepdaughter, Ida Amalie, lifted her hands from the blanket and gave her a coat of red nail polish.

"I know | I don't know | I know | I don't know", she said in English, and I understood it as if she were standing before death, wavering between knowing everything and nothing at all. I had long feared that I would wake up after her death in a panic because she was no longer in the world, but that wasn't the case at all, which is probably because she gave me enough love to be able to live without her. But every now and then I'm consumed with a sudden sorrow that I'll never again hear her voice say my nickname, which was just between me and her, and can therefore only be written here in invisible ink.

25

I meet my father at his front door and we walk over to Holmen's Cemetery together to visit my mother's grave. On the way, he tells me about how the bus line to his winter swimming club has been rerouted, about the architect who designed the new wing of Rigshospitalet, about the painter Magdalene Hammerich's atelier in Lundsgade 9, and he asks if I know who owns the big mansion that's falling apart right on Dag Hammarskjölds Allé, which I don't. "Those are winter tulips", he says, pointing at some little red flowers when we come into the cemetery, "and there are wild tulips growing on the citadel". Grief over the loss of the spouse he knew for seventy-one years and with whom he celebrated a sixty-fifth wedding anniversary hasn't extinguished the old man, who still takes good care of himself and makes sure that he gets outside every day, shops in his neighborhood grocery stores, prepares his own meals, and maintains order in his closet, where his jackets hang in neat rows, and who gets to bed too late every night because he's lost track of time while reading. "If only I can grow old like that", I think. But I'm not him, because, unlike me, he isn't self-absorbed, but is instead absorbed in everything around him. But on the other hand he is also unlike me in that I am writing again, which one hardly does when one's accounts with the world are essentially settled. On the way back we are dazzled by the sight of a flock of black birds high above the lakes, a sharp formation of restless symbols that suddenly dissolve and reassemble into a new, inconceivable configuration.

26

I'd been wanting to write to Mogens Jacobsen for decades to thank him for what he did for my mother, but because she wouldn't have wanted to be reminded of her period of illness, and because if I had written to him anyway it would have felt like going behind her back, it had to wait until she was gone. But Mogens Jacobsen beat her to it and died in 2016, for the past is falling away. Right in front of me.

27

And she especially avoided speaking about the apartment on the fourth floor of Store Kongensgade 23, which my parents sold in 1978 because she associated it with depression. It was likely for the same reason that I moved away from home when I was seventeen to live alone in a rented room out in the city, having lived for just one year at the address that would, conversely, move into me. When you've crisscrossed the lattice of this city's streets as long as I have, you can't avoid passing by places where, many years ago, you ran your once-so-important errands, or, in the window of a second-hand book shop, catching a glimpse of a beat-up book that used to mean so much, while Jethro Tull's "it was a new day yesterday, but it's an old day now" rings in your ears. But then all I have to do is turn the corner and stand in front of Store Kongensgade 23, and the future will begin all over again.

Through the glass panes of the front door I see the checkered terrazzo floor of the entryway, the tall, light-gray wainscotting, and the elegantly swooping banister that winds its way up the building, and then I remember the smells of the paint and the wall-to-wall carpets (strange how we can remember smells) in our new apartment, which we must've traveled from Stevns to take a look at before we moved in, because in my memories it's always so empty that there's plenty of room to dream, not least the dream that I, having won the lottery, might one day reconquer this apartment, which my father bought in 1972 for 200,000 kroner but which now goes for around 8 million whenever it unjustly changes hands between persons unknown.

I'd be in business in those two lovely adjoining rooms that face the street, answering emails and phone calls and playing office at my pinewood desk as, floating majestically over the street, I listened to the ever-rumbling festival of traffic and relished the sight of the sun hitting the gleaming cars that reflect spots of dancing light onto the ceiling. And behind me in the twilit oval corner room I would have my library, where, with my back turned to it all, I could let everything flow toward me from the pages of my books. But at night I would retreat into one of the quiet rooms deep within the apartment, lie in bed, and listen to the blessed sound of autumn rain falling in the courtyard or curl up and sleep like a bear in the dark of winter, only to awake the next morning to a resurrected world.

28

Jane comes to Copenhagen once every summer to visit her family, and then we have dinner and go off in search of one of the smoky old bars that have managed to survive since the '70s. Last time, we sat at one of the tables on the sidewalk in front of Hereford Steak on Store Kongensgade, and we were eating our steaks and getting drunk when she cast a glance across the street. "We're sitting across from *The Address*", she said.

AUTHOR'S NOTE

Thanks to my first readers, Jens-Martin Eriksen and Frederik Stjernfelt.

And to Hans Drachmann, Anne Lise Marstrand-Jørgensen, Jesper Vaczy Kragh, and Raben Rosenberg, to whom I am grateful for providing information for sections 19 and 20 of this book, though naturally this does not necessarily mean that they share my views.

And thanks, as well, to Morten Kirckhoff for the photo series from Oringe.

REFERENCES

Søren Ulrik Thomsen, "Vejen mellem to skoler" ["The Road Between Two Schools"], in *Min skolevej* [*My Way to School*] (Copenhagen: Vindrose, 1989); reprinted in all editions of the *Collected Works of Søren Ulrik Thomsen*, most recently in 2021. Here one can read about the same events as those with which this book is concerned, told thirty-one years prior with other details and other omissions.

Søren Ulrik Thomsen, "Balladen om den tynde mand" ["The Ballad of a Thin Man"], in *Repremiere i mit indre mørke* [*Reprise in My Inner Darkness*] (Copenhagen: Vindrose, 2009); reprinted in all editions of *Collected Works*. In the third section of this poem one can read a more detailed portrait of my father.

Peter Handke, [*A Sorrow Beyond Dreams*], trans. [from German to Danish] Birte Svensson (Copenhagen: Gyldendal, 1976).

Hanne Thomsen, *Et hverdagsliv i 1900-tallet—og andre historier fra familiens liv* [*Daily Life in the 1900s and Other Family Stories*] (privately printed, 2018).

Hanne Thomsen, *Hanne skrev* [*Hanne Wrote*] (privately printed, 2020). Selected poems.

Raben Rosenberg, "Den psykofarmakologiske udvikling 1950–1970" ["Psychopharmalogical Developments, 1950–1970"], in Jesper Vaczy Kragh (ed.), *Psykiatriens historie i Danmark* [*Psychiatry's History in Denmark*] (Copenhagen: Hans Reitzels Forlag, 2008).

Jesper Vaczy Kragh, "'Det er som et mirakel!': Chokbehandling med insulin og cardiazol 1937–54" ["'It's Like a Miracle!': Shock Therapy with Insulin and Cardiazol 1937–54"], in idem, *Psykiatriens historie i Danmark*.

Joanna Moncrieff, *The Myth of the Chemical Cure: A Critique of Psychiatric Drug Treatment* (London: Palgrave Macmillan, 2009).

Einar Geert-Jørgensen, Mogens Hertz, Knud Knudsen, and Kjærbye Kristensen, "LSD-Treatment—Experience Gained Within a Three-Year Period", *Acta Psychiatrica Scandinavica*, November 1964.

Alex Frank Larsen, *De sprængte sind: Hemmelige forsøg med LSD [The Blown Minds: Secret Experiments with LSD]* (Copenhagen: Informations Verlag, 1985).

Andreas Relster, "Medicinen virker ikke, men bivirkninger er gode nok" ["The Medicine Doesn't Work, but the Side Effects Are Pretty Good"], *Information*, 19 September 2009, in which one can read: "Børge Sommer, a health inspector at the Mid-Jutland Regional Hospital, refers to the fact that, since World War II, there has always been 'some drug or other' that doctors have prescribed for psychological problems in the belief that it could solve them. 'First it was holiday pills, and then came the barbiturates, which we probably knew were somewhat dangerous because, if you overdosed on them, you'd die. Which is why we welcomed the widespread adoption of benzodiazepines in the mid-'60s. They were marketed as completely harmless', says Børge Sommer. After fifty years, we are now beginning to realize that, like their predecessors, they [benzodiazepines] are not the solution to all our problems. For Børge Sommer, the big question is whether we will allow history to repeat itself once more, this time with 'happy pills'".

Anne Lise Marstrand-Jørgensen, "Medicin gør det hele værre: Samtale med Janus Christian Jakobsen, overlæge, Copenhagen Trial Unit, Rigshospitalet" ["Medicine Makes Everything Worse: A Conversation with Janus Christian Jakobsen, Superintendent, Copenhagen Trial Unit, Rigshospitalet"], in *En flod skal være i bevægelse: Erindringer og samtaler om angst og depression [A River Must*

Be in Motion: Memories and Conversations about Angst and Depression] (Copenhagen: Gyldendal, 2018).
Psykiatriens dilemma [*Psychiatry's Dilemma*], television documentary, episodes 1–3, DR 2019.

And Hans Drachmann's many articles in *Politiken* about overmedication at the Glostrup Psychiatric Center, including:

Hans Drachmann, "Psykiatri på sprøjten" ["Psychiatry in a Syringe"], *Politiken*, 24 June 2012.
Hans Drachmann and Sebastian Goos, "Årelang overmedicinering" ["Overmedicated for Years"], *Politiken*, 7 October 2012.

TRANSLATOR'S NOTES

Unless otherwise indicated via the citations given below, quotations in the main text of this volume have been translated from the Danish versions that appear in the author's original text.

1 Stéphane Mallarmé, "The entire soul evoked", in *Collected Poems of Mallarmé*, trans. Henry Weinfeld (University of California Press, 2011), 77.

2 The author is quoting here from his poem "Forgive me for seeing your bones before your flesh", the opening lines of which are translated by Susanna Nied as follows: "Forgive me for seeing your bones before your flesh | your flesh before your dress | and your dress before your floating gaze". See Søren Ulrik Thomsen, *Selected Poems*, trans. Susanna Nied (New York: Meeting Eyes Bindery, 1999), 25.

3 The Queen's Court.

4 A humanistic and communitarian institution providing adult education.